MW01228786

Dedication

To My Mother, *Eleanor Dockery*

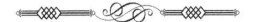

The
AUTISTIC
Child

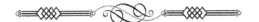

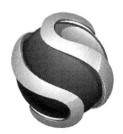

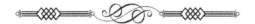

The
AUTISTIC
Child

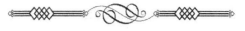

ROBERT LEE DOCKERY

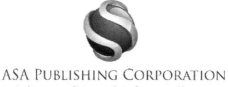

ASA PUBLISHING CORPORATION
AN INNOVATIVE OUTSOURCE BOOK PUBLISHING HYBRID

ASA Publishing Corporation
29 S. Monroe St., Suite 201, Monroe, Michigan 48161
An Accredited Publishing House with the BBB
www.asapublishingcorporation.com

Copyrights©2022, Robert Lee Dockery, All Rights Reserved
Book Title: The Autistic Child
Date Published: 10.15.2022
Book ID: ASAPCID2380863
Edition: 1 *Trade Paperback*
ISBN: 979-8-9868454-6-3
Library of Congress Cataloging-in-Publication Data

This book was published in the United States of America.
Great State of Michigan

Table of Contents

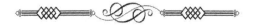

The
AUTISTIC
Child

ROBERT LEE DOCKERY

The Autistic Child

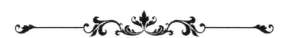

Hi, I am Robert Lee Dockery and I was born on May 23rd, 2001 at Providence Hospital. I was diagnosed with autism at the age of two years old. My mom had noticed that there was something wrong with me because when I was in my infant months, I would say Mama, and suddenly I had stopped saying it. So, my mom had started noticing it more and more when I became of this age. She decided to take me to Grant Preschool to get me checked out to see if I had hearing problems too, because when people would call me I would not respond.

When I was being checked out for it, the testing lady had rattled some keys at me so that I could hear the keys and focus on them. When the test finally came back, they said that I did not have any hearing problems, however, they did diagnose me with Autism since I was not talking. My mom was crying to the people at the Grant Preschool to please help her son. I was the youngest person there at the time to start preschool at the age of 2.

I remember my instructor name Mrs. Marge changing me on the changing table when I used to go to the bathroom on myself, and I even remember her teaching me how to talk by having me use a device that had options like when I needed something to drink, or when I needed something to eat, or when I need ed to use the bathroom, I will point to it and the instructors would do as I requested.

I did not start talking until I was about four or five years old, so when I was mad or frustrated I would scratch people and scream at the top of my voice because I could not express what I had wanted, and I would also bang my head up against the walls out of frustration. When I was a baby and my brother Darnell had told me that he was scared for me, and so was my mom.

One day when I was about four or five years old I have finally said Mama in a loud high-pitched voice, and my mom was so happy she was in tears of joy; my words just started to all come together, it was like a huge accomplishment have been done with me. I was finally being able to talk and express the things that I have wanted to do, and be able to do the things that I wanted to do and not have to get angry because I can't express myself. This led to me to being able to learn things like playing video games and going to Special Ed classes for general education, and how to interact with people, etc.

Back in 2007, I had my first video game system and it was the GameCube. I had games like Sonic the Hedgehog, Madden NFL 2008, GoldenEye 007, Super Smash Mario Brothers, Soulcalibur, Viewtiful Joe, and Pac-Man. I will play these games to try and learn how to play them. And, I am having fun learning how to play them on my period at the Elementary School I was attending. My mom used to be excited for me when I was playing these games because I was learning how to play them well.

I had went to Roosevelt Elementary School for two years; 2007-2009, and the thing that I learned there was how to do math like adding and subtracting numbers and colors, while going to the gross motor room to play and interact with other kids. The instructors, whenever it was time to eat, they would show me options of food and I had to pick which one of them that I had liked.

I remember Mrs. Mary who was one of my instructors at Roosevelt and Kennedy Elementary, she was very instrumental in me having the knowledge that I have to this day. She told me things like 'I will always love you no matter what' and would correct me when I did not listen, or when I said things that were inappropriate. I also remember Mrs. Ansel answer who was also one of my instructors at Roosevelt and Kennedy. She always motivated me to be at my best and she would get on me for not listening to instructions and she always loved me I would. I went to Kennedy Elementary in 2009 to 2010, and when I went there I learned how to interact with kids. This is when I started to go back and forth from General Ed classes to Special Ed classes, and starting to learn things like how to read and do math by reading with the whisper phone, and doing tasks in the morning . . . I'm off.

I can remember back in 2009 to 2010 we would

also go to the pool to learn how to swim, and in 2010 when I had went to a summer day camp called the Recreation Building to also learn how to swim with a lifeguard. Back in 2009 when I got my PSP and the games that I had were God of War, Viewtiful Joe, Madden Smackdown vs Raw 2007, and Grand Theft Auto: Liberty City Stories.

I remember back on my birthday back in 2009 I got up in the morning and we went and had breakfast, and then we went to GameStop to go buy the games that I had wanted. My dad had saw Smackdown vs Raw 2007, he suggested that I get that instead of the Madden game I wanted. He bought Smackdown vs Raw 2007 for me. I was mad and kept saying "I hate wrestling . . . I hate wrestling!" And my dad, he kept saying "Try it Buddy (my nickname is Buddy).

Next, we went home to get ready to go up under the shed. This is a spot that my mom and her friends would always go to hang out at, and the next thing you know my stomach would hurt. I started crying, saying to my mom that my stomach hurts. So, we went up under the bench crying.

The next thing that we did was we went home and my sister Katrina and our cousin Shanell came with us to celebrate my birthday at the house, but I went and laid in the back room, still crying in agony. The next thing you know in a split second, my stomach was feeling a little bit better, and got up and started to play my Smackdown vs Raw 2007 video game for my PSP. I actually began to like it, and as a result I started to have fun with it . . . and I would go on and continue to have lots of fun with this video game.

I remember this one night back in 2010, I had stayed up all night playing this game, and having so much fun playing with all kinds of wrestlers in it and making the wrestlers bleed as their blood would hit the mat in the ring. I would also would have fun doing my finisher with the wrestlers that I was playing with against the computer, and when I had done my finisher on the computer, the computer would lay a knockout kind of posture like he was dead or some with his head busted in pieces. Then, I would go on and pin him and the ref would count one two three, and I had won the matches. It was a glorious moment for me! I will play with wrestlers such as Triple H, John Cena, Mr. Kennedy, Shawn Michaels, and so many more other wrestlers in the game.

My Autistic Special Talents

    I remember this one day back in 2010, I was riding with my mom and I will point out the names of the cars other people were driving. For example; I would say that person is driving a Pontiac or that person is driving a Chevrolet just by looking at the car symbols in the front. My mom was amazed like 'wow how did he even do this and get it right at the same time?' My mom then bought me a Gallagher arcade system on May 23rd, 2020 for my 19th birthday; I was 9 years old. Also, my mom was so proud of me, she would say things like you are so smart because I would see every car riding pass, and I would look at the design of the car and would get some complicated cars right too, for example; if I saw a BMW or a Volkswagen, I would get those cars right by looking at the back them. I also remember back in 2010 when I used to play SmackDown vs Raw 2007 on my PSP, I would just play and teach myself how to play the game without anybody showing me, and got really good at it. When I was playing the game, I would make the wrestler bleed. And when it was time for me to do my finisher with the wrestler that I was playing with, the computer that's playing against me would be knocked out. Then, I would pin the wrestler and the referee would count to three, and I would win the match.

I also remember on my 19th birthday back on May 23rd, 2020, I got a Galaga arcade and a Pac-Man arcade, and when I had started to play I just taught myself how to play it and got really good at the arcade games. For example, on my Galaxy arcade game I just taught myself how to move around and avoid the monsters that came down on me with a single rocket, and I taught myself how to move with the double rocket because when you play with the single rockets, there would be a monster that would trap you in. And if the single rocket got caught in it as well, you would have to shoot the monster to unlock the rocket that was also caught. This would allow you to receive a double rocket to work with. Now, the double rocket moved a lot slower than the single rocket, but it was shooting faster as well. At first, I had a hard time moving with the double rocket because I was figuring out how to avoid all the fast moving monsters, because in the higher stages of the game the monster would come down on you a lot faster than the beginning.

I also taught myself how to become a better shooter with the double rocket as well, by watching a guy on YouTube that played Gallagher. And, what I watched him do was he used the high score at the top to line up his double rocket to shoot the monsters at the top, and he would get the monsters at such an accurate rate. As a result, he did not die until he had reached 270,000 points as his high score on Galaga. I remembered when I first started to play Galaga, I had set my high score to 169,000 and it took me a long time to beat my high score on Galaga because I was trying to practice all the tricks, and learning the complexities of the game. But, for some reason I would come up just short or an inch closer to beating my high score, even though I would get unlucky and die at the last minute because of the fast moving monsters that would get me in the last minute.

This one day that I was playing Galaga back in 2021 before I had went to college, I hopped on it and started firing away with the single rocket first. I was getting the monsters until I had got stuck with one of the them that had trapped me in the corner. And as a result I had lost one of my lives because also when the monster gets your single rocket you lose a life, and then you have to start over on that same level; you have to shoot the monster that has the rocket to unlock the double rocket.

So, I was firing away with a single rocket for a moment and when I had approached the monster that had my rocket, I shot the monster and I got my double rocket. And from there I was shooting the monsters with so much accuracy, that you would think that I was in a shootout with somebody. That's how accurate I was with the double rocket! And, when I was on the bonus stages on Galaga, I would get all of the monsters and would earn a lot of bonus points which would later help me beat my high score on it. In the meantime, I was firing away with the double rocket for a good moment, and when I saw that I had beat my high score to $196,000 on Galaga I have felt so proud of myself; it was like a huge monkey was off my back. When I had told my mom that I had beaten it she was in joy and amazed, thinking 'Wow! Now how did Buddy beat this high score like that?"

I told her how I beat it and she was like 'damn buddy, you are really good at this Gallagher game,' and then she had asked how did I get this good at this Gallagher game? I told her that I taught myself how to play Galaga, by teaching myself how to move with the double rocket, and by shooting all that you can as quick as you can. And, whatever monster is left you go to the high score section of the game and then the monster will approach you on that section. You then move in the corner and keep shooting regardless of where you are at in the game.

And, at the beginning of a new level you just shoot all the monsters the best way you can with the limited mobility of the double rocket to your advantage, and to never get stuck in one place. I also told my mom that she that the single rocket is faster than a double rocket because you can avoid the monster a lot quicker, and you can shoot good but not as good as the double rocket. But I also told my mom that I was just as good with the single rocket as I was with the double rocket.

So, I shot the monster and I had unlocked the double rocket on Galaga, and I was hitting the monsters at an extremely accurate rate, and as a result I was getting higher in the game and I finally beat my high score to $196,000 in the game, and I was so relieved my emotions were also intense. I was feeling so many emotions at once like happy, surprise, Joy, amazed, and proud of my special talents when it came to my game Galaga.

Next, I have beaten my high score to 230,000 in just a few months going through my trials and tribulations in the game, by coming close a few times to coming just short at the last minute because I got hit by the fast moving monsters that was in the game. I remember the day that I had beat the game's high score. I had started off with a single rocket and was hitting the monster with great accuracy and had great mobility as I was avoiding the monsters that would come down on me. I was also avoiding the bullets that was coming down on me from the monster shooting at me at such a fast pace in the game, the next thing you know I got sucked in by the monster that had trap me in the corner and I had to shoot him to earn my double rocket, which I did and as a result on the next level. I was shooting the monsters as fast as I could to avoid having to move around so many monsters because of my limited mobility with the double rocket, and as a result I had less monsters to work with. I was even able to move around with the double rocket a lot easier. This was a method that I had taught myself how to do just then, and I was amazed like wow man, so this is how you do it when you have a double rocket - just shoot as many as you can then you would have an easier time avoiding the monsters because there are less you have to deal with on that particular level.

I just used that same method that I had taught myself on the higher levels, and as a result I was able to get all the monsters in bonus rounds too. There were bonus 1 rounds in the game as well, and the bonus rounds when I had the double rocket I would get all the monsters by remembering all the patterns that the monsters had did. As a result, I got all of the 40 monsters that was in the bonus rounds. There were 40 monsters that were in each bonus round. When I got all 40 monsters in the bonus rounds, I would get a lot of bonus points for getting all of them, and it would make my scores higher. It gave me motivation for the next levels that I had to do that day when I beat my high score.

So when I had got to the stage where I beat my high score, I remember when I was in shock like wow, I beat my high score and I had kept going until I reached 230,000, and I was happy like damn, I have finally beat my high score and I did it with such effort. There was so much tribulation which made it so satisfying for me, because I had went through so much trying to beat my high score in those few months I have played Galaga.

Next, I have beat my high score to $244,000 which is my current high score for now. I'm currently in the process of beating it. I have come close to it, but I came up just short as of now. Next I taught myself how to play this computer game called Snake, and Snake is a game that you control a green snake; there is going to be a red block that the snake has to eat in order for it to grow large.

The Autistic Child

The game moves in a fast pace, and if the red block gets trapped in the corner then you would have to move quick on the dime because if you don't you will hit the wall and die as a result of it, and then you have to start over. Also in the game, the longer the snake grows the more harder it is to find the red block. Get the red block in the game because the snake is so long and the game can sometimes put the red block in some unfavorable positions like in the corner, or inside of your snake, and since the game moves so fast you might hit the wall so easily you'll have to start over again.

I remember back in 2021 in the summertime I would play Snake, and I would go through my trials and tribulations with this game. I had set my high score to 225 at first and I would come close to beating my high score, but I will come up just short at first because I was getting my snake hit by the wall because the red block happened to be there, but I had taught myself now to move quick on the dime so that my snake would not run into the wall. I had also taught myself to follow the tail end of my snake so that I can get the red block easier with the snake getting long, and the game moving faster.

I had also taught myself how to do a zigzag kind of motion with the snake and kind of let the tail end of the snake get closer to the red block and when the snake clears I would get the red block and my snake would grow longer. I remember I had also taught myself how to move quick on the dime if the if the red block was on the wall because the snake will get hit on the wall if you are not quick enough also. I remember I had beat my high score to 269 back in 2021 on this nice hot summer day I was going through trials and tribulations as I was playing Snake. I had kept coming close to beating my high score multiple of times but I came just short until I played it again, and all of a sudden I had clicked on all Snyder's cylinders and I was getting all of the red blocks, and the next thing you know I have beaten my high score on it.

I also played Snake a few months, or so ago, and have beaten my high score to 289 on it, and then beaten my high score on it about a few months later. This is by teaching myself how to do it, like motion while the tail end of the snake was moving and then I had to follow it to get to the red block, and that's how I beat my high score.

The Autistic Child

I also can remember dates very well and my remembrance of them helped me remember certain details of my life very vividly. For example, I can remember the things that happened from like 2007 o up until now because I have lived them, and I paid great attention to detail back then.

And, I can remember the date of the current days very well too. For example, at this job that I am currently working at called the Fox Run. When I would fill out the Covid sheets, there it said today's date I would automatically remember that day's date without looking at my phone or anything because that special talent got better with time because I used to have to look at my phone to check that day's date. I also use this special talent to help my mom remember certain things that she has to do on that specific date, and I do a very good job with it as it helps keep my mom organized and it keeps the stress off her to remember to do things also. I also tell my family members like my sister, brother, aunt, uncles and cousins stuff that I have remembered in the past like for example, I told my Auntie Shirley when we were at my Cousin Mark's baseball game back in 2010.

My mom is always amazed at this special talent as she says wow-wee Buddy that is an amazing special talent that you have, and my Aunt Shirley always said that you are a special guy.

I also taught myself how to play my other arcade game called Pac-Man that I got on my birthday. This is by allowing my Pac-Man to wait in the corner until the monsters came in one spot, and then I ate the big cheese to make them turn blue and would eat them all to get my score higher. I also taught myself to trick the monsters when I had a little bit of cheese left near the end of the levels by going up with the monsters, then down so that the monsters could follow me, then back up again so I could get the cheese that were originally down that same path. Or, I would teach myself to go down when the monsters were up so I could trick them to come down with me, so then I could get the cheese on the top to advance to the next level. I also would teach myself to do a kind of back and forth motion to trick the monsters away, so that I could get the big cheese and then eat them all as fast as I could.

My Special Connection

with Dogs

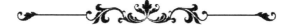

 I remember back in 2009, I would always play with this dog named Zimba, and Zimba was my sister's friend Jordan and Erin's dog. At first Zimba was always aggressive towards me and other people but when I started to be around him, he started to be nice to me and he always even licked me. I remember somebody telling me you just got done playing with that dog. I also remember this one day I was playing with Zimba, Jordan and Erin's granddaddy yelled at me about playing with Zimba, and I think I had stopped playing him after that. I also remember back in 2012, we had got this dog named Oreo, and he was a heavenly dog. At first, it took him a short while to get used to us, but when he did get used to us he loved the s*** out of my mom, and he would bite anybody who messed with my mom. He would go with my mom everywhere she went. Also, I had a good relationship with Oreo, I would play with him and he would lick my feet every time I would go in the basement before I had went to school. Oreo would get aggressive whenever he did not feel like going outside. He was smart as hell. Oreo would knock on the door like he was a human being whenever he wanted to come in the house, and he would stay put in the backyard and never run out.

I remember Oreo would chew my mom's underwear, and my sister's underwear, and they would always get mad when he did this, then we would have to put him outside. Oreo was black and white, that's why we named him Oreo. Oreo would also get aggressive when my mom and dad got into arguments because Oreo felt that he had to protect mom, and my dad will get mad at Oreo. I remember this one day back in 2017, Oreo had rode with my mom to go see about these houses that were on sale, and Oriole had hopped out of the car to go follow my mom and got hit by a car; by a careless driver.

My mom called my sister Katrina and told her that Oreo had just got hit by a careless driver, and she started crying and stuff. At first, my sister Katrina thought my mom was just lying, but my sister had saw that my mom wasn't, and she began getting sad as well. Oreo was a big dog to the family because he provided stability for my mom and us for years, and he was potty trained; never peed or pooped in the house, and he would knock on the door whenever he needed to use the bathroom.

Oreo was a sweet dog to us, man. So, when I found out along with Katrina that the dog really died, it was like my heart had dropped because back then my mom took me and my sister Katrina to school and Oreo was with us, and that was my last time ever seen Oreo again. Man, this s*** still hurts till this day.

I remember back in 2018, we had went to this pet store center and we were looking at dogs and stuff, and we saw this German Shepherd mixed with wolf. My mom and my sister looked at him and they were like wow this dog is cute or whatever. So, my mom decided that she wanted to buy this dog, and so we got him, and we named him Bronco. Bronco was a hyper dog, but he was sweet; he was a strong dog too. Bronco would get on my mom's nerves because he was so hyper and so explorative. Remembering back in 2018, we would take him to dog school to get him trained because he was so active. He had some good days and dog school but he was still hyperactive, so we just gave up on dog school for Bronco.

I remember this one day my sister's boyfriend Jaylin at the time had got rid of Bronco, and he told this person that he got rid of the dog and that Bronco was still a baby at the time, and because he was still hyper.

I remember back in 2020, when my brother had got this dog he named him Carmelo. This was because he is what we call him still, a chilled dog. I remembered my brother Denzel would always bring Mello around when he first got him, and I formed a very special connection with Mello. Mello was a baby at the time back in 2020 when Denzel first got him. Me and Mello clicked off the bat, and I was playing with him and s***. I also used to babysit him whenever my brother Denzel went on the family trips back in 2020, and I would get a chance to really get to know the dog by bringing him over my sister's house. This is because I was going to my sister's house while my family was gone on their family vacation called Put-In-Bay in Ohio, and I had to watch my baby nephew Jayce too at the time. So, I was babysitting and dog sitting at the same time. At first, I was scared to bring the dog in because I was scared he might attack the baby, but my brother said he's not going to do nothing so I just brought him in and I just started to click with Mello automatically; hop on the couch and started to play with me, and he rolled up so I could pet him and stuff. Next, I had took him outside along with my sister's boyfriend at the time with Jaylin's dog named Porsche. And Porsche was a Pitbull who was hyperactive, but she was nice and she would do the same thing Mello did when I came over; rollover so I could pet her.

I remember when my brother's girlfriend had dropped Mello off to us back in 2020 because she needed us to look after him, and I instantly agreed to it because of the bond that I had created with him instantly beforehand, and I had started to really spend time with him since he was really permanently about to stay with us. I remember back in spring 2021, I would start to bring mellow outside with me to go sit on the Porch with me so I could chill with him, and Mello would always stay still with me, and play with me when he felt like playing. Next, he would start to come in with me and would hop on my bed so that he could come lay down with me on my bed while I watch TV. By the way, Mello is a miniature bulldog.

I have spent time with Mello and my other dog Tobi before I had left for the college back in 2021, and I remember mellow would always fight Toby over me, or Toby would fight Mello over me, or vice versa when they would be on the bed together with me. I tried to get them to coexist with each other, but they would not listen to me as their animosity toward each other grew before I had went to college. It was like two jealous brothers going at each other's throat but except they were dogs, and that's when I finally stopped trying with them. And I understood that's how they are. I have bonded with the dogs so much that they were barking at me as they were talking to me, but except it was in their language. Especially, whenever they needed food, and I would go outside to go feed them as was needed, and then they would stop barking because they were satisfied with their food.

I **also bonded** with the dogs so much that if it were to be raining the dogs would bark for me to bring them in, and so I could spend time with them. But, I would bring them in and put them in their cages, and because they were wet from being outside in the rain. They would also bark for me to come and get them early in the morning because they were ready to eat, and when I came to get them, they would take turns rolling over so I come pet each one of them on their tummy. But, when I would get the other dog, I would come pick him up so I could take him outside and feed him food along with Mellow who I also took outside earlier to go eat his food.

As for Toby, the new edition to the family, he is a Shih Tzu mixed with poodle, and I remember when we first got him back in 2019, he was so sweet he could give everybody kisses, and he would play with us because he got used to us very quickly.

My Special Connections With People

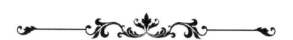

I remember back in 2017 when I was in the 10th grade, I met a guy named Deonte. Me and him had started to click instantly as we're talking about things in my 10th grade English class. The stuff we were also talking about were stuff that made us mad about this football team called the Detroit Lions. They were a team that had a history of losing out. However, they were doing pretty good this time around, so we had talked about how the coach who was Jim Caldwell at the time, had needed to be a little bit more passionate about his job like the head coaches on other teams. For example, this coach named Pete Carroll who was the head coach for this team called the Seattle Seahawks at the time was a very passionate coach, and he would fire up his players before game so that they can be passionate to play. The next, thing I know, I ended up getting his number, and we started to get to know some more stuff about each other, like what foods that he and I like to eat. And, I got to know that he liked basketball too, so we continued talking about how he liked the sport from back in 2012 and in the 2013 era, where Lebron James used to play for the heat and Carmelo Anthony used to play for the Knicks. So, we had so much fun talking about those things that I remembered from that time era too. For example, I had told him about the time that between the Miami Heat and the San Diego Spurs with my dad, and when my dad had saw that the Miami Heat had won, my dad was mad like "That's some Hollywood ass bullshit, man!" because the LeBron James led the super team at the time.

Next, he would talk about more personal things like how he was poor and the trial and tribulations that he had went through; like when he was homeless at one point and he had to spend nights at churches and stuff. He talked about the anger he felt living poor, and I told him that if he ever needed me for anything he can call me because I know the feeling of not having anything, and the anger that it creates on people. So as a result, when we linked up for school at lunchtime, I would look out for him and buy him a cookie or something, to show that I care and understood on what it was like. I said it the best way that I could at the time. Next I had eventually asked him could he ask his mom to see if I could spend the night over there, but Dante said that his parents did not allow company over back in 2020, because the Covid outbreak had just hit so strong and hard around the nation, and I respected that.

Well, I just continued to be there for him as a listing ear, and to call up and check on him from time to time; to make sure he's doing okay. Also, me and Dante went back to talking about goals that we have met in our lives. For example, Dante had wanted to show me stocks that his uncle is doing, and he told me when he gets his car and driver's license he was going to show me those stocks because I had looked it up for him in his time of need, and I'm still doing so as of 2022.

Dante has showed me the car that he had bought

for himself back in 2021 when I was in grade college, and the car was a red Pontiac. It felt like a huge accomplishment for Dante because of what he had went through to get to this stage in his life.

Me and him had always talked about him getting his car, and learning how to drive so that we can hang out together and make money together. We also talked about how I could learn how to drive since I already had my own car, so that we could maybe race each other in each of our cars, and if his were to break down I got him on a ride to go wherever he wanted to go. We also talked about him getting his license, but it was always something; whether it was the weather, or it was his circumstances at home, or whatever. I'm just giving him his time to get it together so that we can get started on our goals. I also used to spend a lot of time with him when we was going to school, and the school that we went to was Ferndale Middle School and High School. They were connected together, and the stuff that we did was when in the Commons at lunch time. And, we went to the courtyard sometimes, but we mainly just sat at the lunch table talking about football and what happened in the classes that we were in together or not in together, and also talking about the teachers having a great time with each other.

After school, we would just hang out on our spare time before our parents called us to tell us that they were here to pick us up, and we would then pick it back up the next day in school. Also, we would be each other's partners in school projects whenever a project came along in the classes that we had with each other. And in those projects that we had with each other we did so well because we were both smart as hell, and we would always come up with good ideas for them. It was like we were Shaq and Kobe, the way that the ideas were flowing at the time between us. In school we would also talk about serious issues like mass shootings, dumb things people did in Detroit and still doing, and sobriety - being a straight edge, and we would also talk about these things over the phone as well, then and now in 2022. I also remember this one conversation that we had a few months ago that we had about both of our special talents, and we talked about how he can draw; learning things very quickly remember things, etc.

My Autistic Challenges in School and How I Overcame Them

   I remember back in 2010 to 2011 when I was in the elementary school; it was Kennedy Elementary that I went to. When I was there, I used to jump up and down because I was hyperactive in school and the teachers used to always tell me to breathe in and out because that's what they knew would calm me down for a bit. But, I would always do it for like a second, and then get right back to jumping up and down like it was nothing. Also, I would always rock back and forth in my chair; back then too, and my ParaPro would always tell me to sit still, but I did not listen. This continued on for the majority of the time that I had went to elementary school, and this led to the teachers yelling at me. I would always cry because my feelings were hurt. For example, when I was in elementary school back in 2013, I was sitting next to my friend Al-Quadeer and was rocking back and forth in my chair, and my teacher at the time, Mr. Williamson had yelled at me for rocking back and forth. The next thing you know I had started crying and telling my resource teacher who had helped me in elementary school from 2010 to 2014, Mrs. Adamson that Mr. Williamson had yelled at me for rocking back and forth in my chair, and Mrs. Adamson had talked to Mr. Williamson about it and Mr. Williamson had said that he was sorry and that he had been frustrated that day. Also, my sister Katrina had got on me about rocking back and forth in my chair back then too. She used to yell at me for rocking back and forth too, but I would rebel against her and tell her things like I can do what I want to do in school and you are not the boss of me, and stuff like that.

My mom would get on me about rocking back and forth in my chair also, but I did not listen. So as a result, back in 2013, she had took me to the development center to see if there was anything wrong with me, and the doctor had diagnosed me with ADHD. I then had to start taking medication for this so that I could sit still in school, but I did not want to take the medication. So, my mom used to force me to take the it, so I did.

I remember back in 2013, I also won *Student of the Week* for in Mrs. Watson's class, she was my teacher at the time for being good in class and staying focused and doing my assignments. I told my mom that I had won the award, and she told me the reason that I had one the award was because I had took my medication like I was supposed to. But I did not believe this at the time, and I did not want to take my medication during that time, neither. But my mom made me take it before I had went to school.

Also, Mrs. Watson would yell at me for rocking back and forth in my chair and for talking when I was not supposed to be. This would hurt my feelings a lot back in 2012 to 2013, but Mrs. Watson would always say that she's sorry, but this is the way that she will be with me. That I am going to have to behave and sit still in my chair in her classroom and not talk when I am not instructed to. And as a result, I would tell the principal on her and the principal, Mr. Adams at the time, would tell me the same thing like you are going to have to learn how to not get mad when people are frustrated with you. But I still did not listen and kept telling him about it, but it was to no avail.

I remember when I was in Middle School back in 2014 to 2015, I had grown out of rocking back and forth in my chair and I noticed myself paying attention to things better, and had started to sit still in my chair. I also had stopped taking medication for ADHD back in 2014, a little before I started Middle School. It was like a huge accomplishment that had just been taken a step forward because I made so much progress back then to the point that I did not need the medication anymore. And as a result, I knew what the teachers were talking about because I wasn't so fidgety anymore, and I could learn more.

My sister had asked me did I still rock back and forth in my chair back in 2015, and I told her no and she was like 'good you need to sit down and focus in school.' Next, I told my mom that I did not rock back and forth from school anymore, and she was very amazed that I had stopped doing it as well. She was so proud of me, it was like a huge accomplishment on her part because she had been trying for years to get me to stop rocking in my chair through taking me to doctors and having my sister Katrina tell me to stop, etc.

I felt really proud of myself for finally being able to sit still in the chair and focus like my other peers in the classroom. Being able to sit still there was another challenge that I had to overcome in Middle School, back in 2014 to 2015. And that challenge was getting my grades up and being able to turn in my assignments.

I remember back in 2014 when I was in LRC class at the time (LRC stands for Learning Resource Center), and my teacher at the time was Mr. Huff who was a big old fat guy and he had called the students up so the students could see their grades on his website called MyStar. So, the next thing you know he calls me up and I saw my grades and they were bad. I had 4- E's, 2- C's, and I think 1- A. The classes that I had the 4- E's in were History, Science, English, and Math. I had the 1- E in LRC, and the 1- A in Art. The teacher has showed me all of the missing assignments that were on the computer, I was so hurt because I thought I was doing so well turns out I was doing so s******. But I did not know it until he has showed me the grades I had. The next thing you know my math teacher Mr. Phou at the time had given the students their MyStar password so that they could check their grades frequently, and this was when I started to teach myself how to keep track of my assignments and study for quizzes and test, since quizzes and tests were like 75 to 80% of our grade at the time.

Soon, I had gradually started to get my grades up in school and paying attention to the teachers and asking for help when I had needed it, and as a result I had started to do well on my test and quizzes in classes like Math, English, Science and History. For example, in my History class Mr. Jeffrey my teacher would do a study guide, and he would say you can use the test to help you pass the test, but at first I did not know it as I had put away the study guide just took the test and I always used to fail the test until I heard this. Then, I started to use my study guide to help me pass the test, and as a result I had started to pass these tests at a higher rate, and it became a habit. That I eventually taught myself, and as another result the next trimester I had a better grade in the class.

Another example was in Science. I had taught myself how to study for things by reading things out loud to myself over and over again so that I could pass the quizzes and test. Also, I had taught myself how to keep track of my assignments by checking my grades more so I know that know what specific assignment that I am missing so I could turn it to the teacher to get my grade up in the class. And, I had started to do this for all of my classes. As a result from all this, I got better grades the next two trimesters in Middle School.

The middle school that I went to was Ferndale Middle/High School, they were connected. Soon after, I had started to do well the next year in 8th grade back in 2015 to 2016, but unlike the year before when I had got off to a tough start had out finished strong toward the ending of the 7th grade back in 2014 to 2015.

See, I had came out of the gate on fire as I had already knew what it took to get really good grades in middle school. Now, I would get A's and B's in my classes because I had studied a lot more and I used the motivation from the year before too; stayed buckled and focused on my schoolwork. Also, I started to talk to people less and checked my grades more frequently so that I could see my missing assignments.

The next thing you know, the teachers would always say that I was doing really good work in school, but there was another challenge that I had to overcome and that was my handwriting which I had struggled with throughout my elementary school career, and middle School career. For example, my handwriting was so bad that my sister Katrina would tell me that I needed to start writing like my ParaPro. At that time, it was Miss Angel. Her handwriting back when I was in elementary school was so neat and organized. When I was in Middle School, my sister Katrina would see my assignments when I got home and she would get on me about writing neater so that other people could see my work. My mom would also get on me about my handwriting, and she would say things like 'you need to write neater so that other people can see your handwriting.'

I also had tried other methods when I was in the 8th grade like maybe writing the words a little bigger on a line piece of paper. I remember one day I had showed her, and she had said, "Buddy why are you writing so big on a piece of paper? This is not how you write," and as a result, I tried writing smaller on a piece of paper but it was to no avail.

I remember back in 2017 when I was in my teacher Mrs. Maes class for physics, I had just started to notice a big change in my writing as everything just started to come together for me in this aspect. My words started to appear neater on a piece of paper, and I started to get compliments on my handwriting later on in my high school career. My sister also has started to notice the change in my handwriting, she would say that I came a long way and that she was so proud of me for overcoming this challenge that I have faced practically my entire life. At this point, I was in the ninth grade at this time, my mom had also seen my improvements in this aspect and she was so proud of me for writing neater on a piece of paper, too. I was so proud of myself for making this huge improvement even though it was later down the road in my school career.

So my lifelong struggle that I had was that I would always read out loud to myself without reading in my head. My entire school career and this led to other kids making jokes like 'damn, you about to read to the entire class' and teachers getting frustrated with me, because reading out loud was the only way that I could learn. For example, I was reading out loud all the time back when I was in a 6th grade in 2013 to 2014, and this one day I was reading because it was reading time, and Mrs. Zold my sixth grade teacher at the time yelled at me to read in our heads. My feelings were hurt and I had cried my eyes out, and the next thing you know Mrs. Zold had told me very kindly that she wanted me to be a better reader. So, that made me feel better and I try to read in my head, but it was to no avail.

I also remember when they used to give me the whisper phones so that I could whisper read to myself. This worked for a minute, but I would gradually start whispering the words to myself 'very loudly to myself', which let me going right back to reading out loud to myself. In high school this would become an issue as kids in my class would say 'damn stop reading out loud like this or they would say 'damn you're about to read to the whole class.' As a result I would have to go outside to go read out loud to myself, and I'd like to do this in high school as it gave me some alone time to read whatever book I was reading, so that I could really learn what the book was about. I also remember when the teachers would always tell me to be quiet and I would try to be quiet, but I would always find myself reading out loud to myself as I could not help this. As of 2022, I have overcome this challenge as I now know how to read in my head, and I can now read with my eyes now.

I also remember back when I was an elementary school and middle school, high school and in college I had struggled to be social with people. For example, back in middle school I had struggled to be social because I was so focused on getting my school work done that I did not think that I had time to be social with other people, when I have my work I had to do. As a result, people thought that I was weird and this let people go behind me doing things like touch my hair when I had started to have my dreadlocks in my hair, back in 2016. These types of things were happening to me because they were wondering why I wasn't social with people. I also was not very involved in the school activities, like going to the dances and the homecomings that they had back then. Back in

2019, I had told my sister that I was not going to homecoming and she told me that I needed to be more social and go to it. "How you think you going to get some girls?"

It had ended up raining that night, so I had told my sister and she said to see if it's going to be raining all night. I had looked it up on my phone and I think it said that it was gone rain all night, so I decided not to go to homecoming that night. I also used to skip homecoming to watch football on that weekend because that was more fun to me than going to homecoming. I also did not socialize with people at lunch before I met someone back in 2017. I used to sit at lunch by myself eating, and when I went to college back in 2021 I did not used to be social, I used to be in my room playing video games most of the time and studying for the next quiz that I had the next day for school. That's what I really cared about at the time. Also, I was really quiet at lunch time as I had a lot going on mentally at the time, and I did not really care to share it at the time. I thought it would be best to keep it private.

I have overcome these things somewhat as I

have made some good friends over the years by the likes of Deonte and my good friend Najae Harris who I met in college. These people are those who have impacted my life in a positive way. And for example, one day I met my good friend Najae Harris in college, we immediately clicked through our football talks, and we used to play Madden 22 a lot in my dorm room. I used to always beat him in it; usually by blowout, but I would always have fun playing with him and he would always have fun playing with me. We would run it back up if we were available.

I also met my friend, Jalen Savage when I was in high school. We would play video games together online with my other friends; Kevin, Deonte, Amari, Matthew, etc. We would have a lot of fun playing Call of Duty and Modern Warfare. I would usually be near last place playing, but I had a lot of fun spending time with them. And in college I met the sweetest girls named, Amari and Anya. They would always help me out if I needed somebody to study with, or if I just needed somebody to talk to. I always appreciate it, and this helped me out a lot when it came down to my mental health. I also met this one girl named Marian-Lynn, and she was a helpful classmate that's spent hours with me to make sure that I had did well on my test, and she was instrumental in helping me pass my great final without her I would not be where I am today.

You have to overcome challenges in life to be successful, and there are many more obstacles to overcome in this lifetime.